Anti-Aging Skincare Explained

Real Talk about What Works, When to use it and which at-home devices are worth your time. No more Confusion!

Contents

For My Mother

Thank you for being my proofreader, Editor-In-Chief, and, as always, my biggest cheerleader. Your wit and wisdom have molded me my entire life.

143

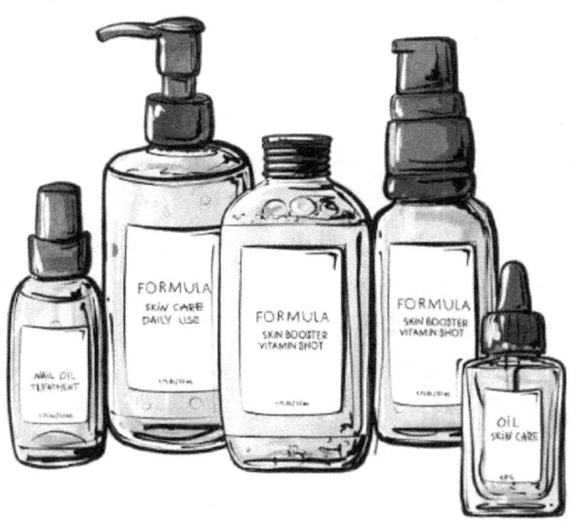

Introduction

Hello, beautiful you!

Imagine You're standing in the skincare aisle of your favorite store. Bright lights shine down on the promises enshrined in glossy packaging, each box a pledge to erase wrinkles, restore radiance, and deliver youth in generous dollops. You're armed with a credit card and a shopping list longer than your last tax return, scribbled from hours of scouring the Internet, poring over beauty magazines, and half-watching morning show segments with celebrity dermatologists. But as you stand there, you can't shake the feeling of being utterly lost in a sea of options. This, my friends, is the skincare paradox, and it's the first thing that we're going to unravel together.

Three years ago, that was me: overwhelmed, under-informed, and ripe for the marketing. I had a bathroom cabinet overflowing with half-used products. A mirror that threw back all my insecurities and sinking feeling that I was playing a game I couldn't win. Spoiler alert: I couldn't win it because I didn't understand the rules. That's what led me down the rabbit hole of skincare science, past the buzzwords and beyond the influencers' raves.

Now, after more trials (and errors) than I can count, it's time to share the honest tea. This book isn't just a compilation of skincare tips: it's the heartfelt account of how I learned to navigate the labyrinth of anti-aging solutions without losing myself (or *all* of my savings). It's about cutting through the noise, understanding what's what, and making informed choices that celebrate our skin rather than wage war against it.

Why should you listen to me? Because I've been where you are, and I've emerged with insights stripped free of commercial whispers. I dove deep so you wouldn't have to, experimenting on myself, interrogating experts, and even throwing myself into the bewildering world of skincare forums where acronyms like AHA and PHA are spoken like a second language.

In these pages, we'll debunk myths and reveal truths. You'll learn why some ingredients are skincare royalty and how to use them wisely. We'll decode the fine print on your favorite products and unveil the at-home devices that genuinely deserve a spot on your vanity. From understanding collagen's real deal to the sunscreen gospel, nothing is off-limits.

But more than that, this journey reclaims the joy of skincare from the jaws of confusion. Remember, this isn t about 'fixing' ourselves – because darlin', we're not broken. It's about feeling empowered and informed to make decisions that enhance our natural beauty at any age. It's self-care that feels like a treat, not a chore.

Expect laughter, 'aha' moments, and maybe a few 'wish I'd known that sooner' groans. Because, let's be honest, who hasn't fallen for a product just because it came in a pretty bottle at least once? Together, we'll navigate this comical pilgrimage, your hand in mine, with all the honesty of a night out with your trusty best friend.

What's to come is a transparent, sometimes cheeky, always enlightening expedition into what it means to age gracefully today. And it's not about recapturing the skin of our 20s but celebrating the journey our skin has been through. Wrinkles? They're a testament to our life lived. Laugh lines? Wear 'em with pride and a wink of your eye! They deserve nothing but the best, and also, they need to slow down a bit, right?

As we delve into the chapters ahead, remember that every piece of advice and each insight comes from a place of love, experience, and a hefty dose of reality. There will be no airbrushing the facts here. And while we're all in for rediscovering that youthful glow, it's more about reigniting the light inside, the one that beams out when you feel good about yourself.

So, if you're ready to step away from the skincare roulette wheel, I'm here to be the friend who takes you aside and says, "Okay, here's what you really need to know." No fluff, no fear-mongering, just fun and facts.

Now, as we transition from this heart-to-heart, we venture into the realm of 'Ingredients that Matter.' It's the bedrock of everything that follows, setting the stage for smarter, savvier, and more effective skincare choices. Ready to flip the script on anti-aging and rewrite it in your own words? Great, let's dive into the nitty-gritty of ingredients, and oh, it's going to be a game-changer!

Chapter 1

INGREDIENTS THAT MATTER

Alright, my savvy skincare companions, it's time to dive into the heart of the matter—the stuff that makes our beloved creams, serums, and magic potions dance to the tunes of rejuvenation and vitality. We're talking about the powerhouse ingredients that make a real difference. No more falling for exotic blends or fancy names that sound like they belong in a sci-fi movie. We're about to break down the who's who of skincare ingredients, and trust me, it's like finding the VIP list for the best anti-aging party in town.

Retinoids (Vitamin A derivatives):

Let's unravel the mystery of Retinol and its close relatives, Retinaldehyde and Tretinoin. Picture a family gathering where everyone is related but each has their unique quirks. That's these three for you, all part of the retinoid family but with distinct personalities in the skincare world.

Retinol is the over-the-counter darling you've seen in all sorts of skincare products. Think of Retinol as the gateway member of the family, potent enough to reduce the signs of aging but generally well-tolerated by most. It works its magic slowly and steadily, boosting cell turnover and collagen production, thereby reducing the appearance of fine lines, wrinkles, and age spots over time. It's your reliable, go-to friend for a rejuvenated complexion without requiring a prescription.

Examples:
The Ordinary Retinol 0.5% in Squalane
CeraVe Resurfacing Retinol Serum
Paula's Choice 1% Retinol Booster

Retinaldehyde is the middle child, if you will. More potent than Retinol but less so than Tretinoin, it's that happy medium for those who need a bit more oomph but aren't quite ready for the heavy hitters. Retinaldehyde is closer to Tretinoin in the conversion process (oh yes, our skin converts these ingredients into something it can use). It typically works faster than Retinol, bringing quicker results with less irritation than its stronger sibling. It's perfect for the "I want results, but I also love my skin barrier" individuals.

Examples:
Maelove Moonlight Retinal Super Serum
Medik8 Crystal Retinal 1 Serum
Avene RetrinAL 0.1 Intensive Cream

Tretinoin is the powerhouse. Available by prescription, Tretinoin is the Hulk of the retinoid family, directly active as soon as it hits the skin, with no need for conversion. It's a favorite for dermatologists tackling severe acne, deep wrinkles, and significant photodamage. But with great power comes...you guessed it, greater potential for irritation. Tretinoin doesn't mess around, so it's the path for those who need serious results and are willing to play the long game, enduring some dryness, flaking, and sun sensitivity (extra caution with the SPF, please).

(Special note - try not to mix Tretinoin with a Glycolic body lotion and use it on your inner thighs. This is bad.)

Each of these retinoids can be a game-changer depending on your skin's needs and tolerance. They're the time-travelers of skincare, turning back the years, but they demand respect. Always ease them into your routine, listen to your skin's feedback, and prepare for progress towards transformation. And remember, patience is key here; these ingredients work their magic over time, not overnight!

Alpha Hydroxy Acids (AHAs):

Ready to exfoliate the confusion away? Let's wade into the world of AHAs, starting with the trio of Glycolic Acid, Lactic Acid, and Mandelic Acid. Imagine them as a team of renovators for your skin, each bringing their own set of tools to the job. Best used as leave-on treatments, they work by ungluing the bonds holding the outer layers of dead skin cells from the healthier, smoother skin beneath.

Glycolic Acid is the best-known and most-researched AHA. Think of it as the speedster, penetrating your skin quickly due to its small molecular size. It sweeps away dead skin cells like nobody's business, revealing a fresher, smoother surface. It's fantastic for a range of issues from acne to aging, but a word of caution: the same properties that make it effective can also make it a tad irritating for sensitive skin. It's the powerful, no-nonsense friend who kicks doors down but sometimes doesn't realize their own strength.

Examples:
CeraVe Skin Renewing Nightly Exfoliating Treatment
L'Oreal RevitaLift DermIntensives 10% Pure Glycolic Acid Serum
Mario Badescu Glycolic Acid Toner

Lactic Acid is a gentler AHA. Its larger molecule size means it's slower to get down into your skin, offering a kinder, more moisturizing approach to exfoliation. If you can imagine a soothing spa day, then that's Lactic Acid for you. It helps you shed those unwanted dead cells while also pulling in moisture where it's needed most. Ideal for sensitive skin types, it's like the friend who brings you soup when you're feeling under the weather - reliable, comforting and leaves you feeling better than before.

Examples:
The Ordinary Lactic Acid 10% + HA 2%
Paula's Choice Advanced Smoothing Treatment

Mandelic Acid, the big buddy in this group, has a large molecular structure, meaning it takes its sweet time getting through the skin's surface. Translation? This big baby causes even less irritation. But don't mistake its gentle nature for ineffectiveness. Mandelic Acid is a warrior against acne, pigmentation, and aging, particularly respectful of sensitive skin and darker skin tones due to its slow and steady nature. It's like that friend who doesn't rush you, understands your pace, and still helps you arrive where you want to be.

Examples:
Naturium Mandelic Topical Acid 12%
Vivant Skin Care 8% Mandelic Acid 3-in-1 Serum

The INKEY List Mandelic Acid Treatment

Choosing between these AHAs is like picking a favorite dance style. They all move to the same rhythm of exfoliation but step differently based on your skin's tempo. Whether you need the fast-paced zest of Glycolic, the balanced rhythm of Lactic, or the slow, soulful sway of Mandelic, you're orchestrating a routine that sings harmony to your skin's unique needs.

Vitamin C:

In the realm of skincare, Vitamin C is the heralded multitasker, known for its brightening, anti-aging, and all-round hero properties. But not all Vitamin Cs are created equal. Let's spotlight two primary forms: Tetrahexyldecyl Ascorbate and L-Ascorbic Acid.

Tetrahexyldecyl Ascorbate is a lipid-soluble form of Vitamin C, ideal for sensitive skin, easily absorbing into deeper layers due to its fat compatibility. It's user-friendly, less prone to causing irritation, and integrates well with other skincare ingredients. Notably stable, it resists degradation from environmental exposures, prolonging the product's effectiveness. However, while it's kinder on the skin and benefits from deeper absorption, it doesn't offer the same intensity in skin brightening and collagen production as its water-soluble counterparts.

Examples:
DRMTLGY's Vitamin C5
Platinum Skin Care's High Octane Vitamin C Serum

L-ascorbic acid stands out as the pure, unadulterated form of Vitamin C, highly acclaimed for its potent effects. This powerhouse ingredient promises vivid brightness and a significant reduction in aging signs and pigmentation, akin to the vibrant intensity of the summer sun. Being water-soluble, it acts promptly at the skin's surface, efficiently neutralizing free radicals and addressing skin damage with remarkable agility, akin to a dependable friend who springs into action without hesitation.

However, it does come with its quirks. L-Ascorbic Acid demands particular care, as it's prone to rapid degradation when exposed to light and air, necessitating special storage considerations like dark-colored, air-tight bottles or tubes. Additionally, its strong personality might not mesh well with all skincare ingredients, necessitating careful formulation pairing. A word of caution as well: due to its high potency, L-Ascorbic Acid may prove too intense for sensitive skin, posing a risk of irritation.

Examples:
Timeless 10% Vitamin C + E Ferulic Acid Serum
LaRoche Posaune 10% Pure Vitamin C Face Serum

In essence, choosing between Tetrahexyldecyl Ascorbate and L-Ascorbic Acid comes down to your skin's personality. Are you looking for a low-fuss, gentle approach with slower, steadier results? Or are you after the most potent punch, provided you can manage a diva's specific needs? Your skincare routine, your call!

Sodium Hyaluronate/Hyaluronic Acid:
Sodium Hyaluronate/Hyaluronic Acid: Within the hydration realm, Sodium Hyaluronate and Hyaluronic Acid are akin to pow-

erful siblings, able to absorb 1,000 times their weight in water. They have similar traits but distinct personalities. Here's how they stack up against each other, considering their superpowers and potential Achilles' heels.

Sodium Hyaluronate:

Think of this as the nimble sibling, a salt derivative of Hyaluronic Acid, smaller in size but mighty in traversing the skin's deeper layers. It's like a hydration ninja, sneaking moisture into the fortress of your skin. Its superpower lies in its ability to hold moisture in those layers, promoting elasticity and resilience against environmental aggressors. However, it's not all smooth sailing. While it's a hydration powerhouse, it doesn't always play the hero for everyone. Some may experience redness or irritation, especially if sensitive to certain salts. It's essential to do a patch test to ensure your skin rallies with this hydrator.

Hyaluronic Acid (HA):

The more renowned sibling, HA is celebrated for its moisture-binding ability, holding water close to the skin's surface, plumping it up like a cushion of freshness. The immediate effect? A visibly hydrated, dew-kissed complexion that feels as luxurious as it looks. Yet, there's a caveat. In arid climates, HA might pull moisture from the deeper layers of your skin instead of the atmosphere, potentially leaving your skin more parched. It's like a well-meaning gardener who unintentionally waters the weeds, too. Additionally, some folks might find it sits on their skin, giving a temporary plump look without long-lasting hydration.

In the end, it's about synergy and balance. Using both types in tandem could offer comprehensive hydration, but awareness of your skin's needs and environmental factors is vital. Consider pairing with other moisturizing agents to ensure HA doesn't backtrack on its hydration promise. Try introducing one new product at a time to catch any unwelcome reactions.

Examples:

Um, literally everything in the skincare aisle

Ceramides and Peptides:

Imagine your skin as a brick wall: ceramides are the mortar holding everything together, while peptides are the messengers, ensuring the wall is well-maintained and robust. Both are vital in the grand scheme of your skin's health and appearance, yet they play very different roles.

Ceramides are the sentinels in your skin's barrier, the lipid molecules that seal the space between skin cells to prevent moisture loss and protect against environmental aggressors. They keep your skin hydrated, pliable, and happy, ensuring no cracks in the fortress. When you apply ceramides topically, you're essentially applying 'reinforcements' to any weak spots in your skin's barrier. It's akin to patching up the gaps in a fence, maintaining a robust barrier against external irritants, and locking in moisture for supple, hydrated skin. The result? Smooth, firm, and hydrated skin that's resilient against environmental onslaughts. They are indeed a boon for dry, sensitive, or eczema-prone skin, working to restore balance and tranquility.

Peptides, on the other hand, are like the skin's local communication network. These short chains of amino acids are the building blocks of proteins, including collagen, elastin, and keratin, which are responsible for the skin's texture and strength.

They're whisperers, signaling your skin to repair itself, encouraging collagen production, and reminding it to spring back into action against the signs of aging. Imagine them as motivational coaches, encouraging your skin to remain robust, elastic, and youthful. The beauty of peptides lies in their gentle nature, making them suitable for sensitive skin. They can help with wrinkles, restore elasticity, and even have a role in healing wounds. Their versatility makes them a worthy ally in various skincare battles.

While ceramides are the guardians of your skin's barrier, peptides are the messengers maintaining the skin's vitality. Incorporating both into your skincare routine can mean a powerhouse of reinforcements, offering a protective shield and proactive repair system, working in tandem to maintain the skin's youthfulness, strength, and resilience.

Examples:
DRMTLGY's Peptide Night Cream
Paula's Choice Barrier Repair Advanced Moisturizer
CeraVe Skin Renewing Night Cream

.

Niacinamide (Vitamin B3):
It's time to zero in on a skincare superhero: Niacinamide, one of the most versatile and mild-mannered ingredients you could introduce to your skin. It's like the friend who brings a toolbox to help fix everything at your house - only this time, it's for your skin.

Here's how it works: For starters, Niacinamide takes on acne by balancing oil production, not aggressively, but like a calm problem-solver. It's effective without causing a scene.

Regarding your skin barrier, think of Niacinamide as the trusty neighborhood watch. It strengthens your skin's defenses, keeping the bad stuff out and the good stuff in. Hydration stays, irritants stay away.

In the anti-aging department, Niacinamide promotes collagen, but it's not about unrealistic standards; it's about supporting your skin's natural charm and strength. It helps keep things smooth, firm, and, yes, naturally youthful.

Hyperpigmentation? Niacinamide is on it, acting like a peacekeeper for your complexion. It addresses dark spots and unevenness, encouraging a harmonious, even skin tone.

Also, this ingredient is your ally against environmental damage. It stands up to the elements and free radicals, like that one community member who's always advocating for a cleaner neighborhood.

The beauty of Niacinamide lies in its compatibility. It gets along with other ingredients and suits almost all skin types, rarely causing issues. In short, it's reliable, kind, and works tirelessly to keep your skin at its best, making your skincare routine less complicated and more effective.

Examples:
Neutrogena Hydro Boost +10 Niacinamide Serum
The INKEY List Super Solutions 20% Niacinamide Serum
COSRX The Niacinamide 15 Serum

Growth Factors:

Alright, let's cut right to the chase and demystify these guys: growth factors are your skin's backstage crew, crucial for keeping everything youthful and harmonious. They're like diligent messengers and overseers within your body. They're there every second, making sure your skin cells do what they need to, like repairing damage and creating new collagen, elastin, or other vital skin components. These proteins naturally occur in your body and are essential for regulating cell growth, helping to repair wounds, restore balance, and rejuvenate the skin on a cellular level - but like everything else, they diminish as we age. *sigh*

Here's when you definitely want these guys on your side:

1. Post-skin procedures or injuries. They're the recovery experts, reducing downtime and tackling scarring like pros.

2. Fighting the signs of aging. Our natural supply drops as we age, so bringing in extra thorough skincare helps smooth out those wrinkles and firm things up.

3. Everyday skincare routine. GFs aren't just for emergencies; using them daily keeps your skin firm, resilient, and glowing.

So, growth factors? They're the negotiators, peacekeepers, and strategists in the world of skincare, working non-stop to keep your skin at its best. Whether it's healing faster or daily maintenance, they're essential for healthy, youthful skin. Bottom line: you want them.

Examples:

The INKEY List 15% Vitamin C + EGF Serum ($)

RevivSerums Ultimate Serum ($$/$)

Skin Medica TNS Advanced+ Serum (not enough room on the page $$$$$$, but the 'Holy Grail)

Broad-Spectrum Sunscreens:

Unless the moon is in the middle of the night sky - YOU MUST WEAR SUNSCREEN. Everyday. All the time. Do Not Fail. And for heaven's sake, don't neglect your neck, chest, arms, hands...

Seriously, nearly 80% of facial aging is due to UV exposure, so we must be diligent.

Okay, the rant is over. Now let's break it down:

Broad-spectrum sunscreens are your ultimate allies against the stealthy impacts of the sun, providing a defense strategy against a whole spectrum of UV rays that cause skin aging and increase cancer risk. Think of them as your skincare bodyguards.

Here's a closer look at the two types:

Physical Sunscreens (Mineral): These guys are like protective outerwear for your skin. Ingredients such as zinc oxide and titanium dioxide form a literal barrier, bouncing off the sun's rays. They're a blessing for sensitive skin types, immediately effective, and less likely to cause breakouts. Plus, they're long-lasting. However, they can leave a chalky cast, making a seamless blend quite the task, especially for richer skin tones. There are beautifully formulated mineral sunscreens with a tint to offset the cast, so try a few and find your favorite.

Chemical Sunscreens: Imagine these as spies who absorb into your skin and neutralize UV rays, turning them into harmless heat. They're the incognito protectors, disappearing on the skin without leaving a trace, making them more appealing for daily use and under makeup. But, a heads-up: they might not be the best buddies for sensitive skin, sometimes causing irritation due to the heat they generate. And by that, I mean they can irritate the devil out of my eyes! I mean - your eyes.

So, why does all this matter? Both types do the heavy lifting in protecting your skin, but they do so differently. The mineral ones sit on top of your skin, deflecting rays, while the chemical versions absorb them before they can do any harm.

Your decision between the two boils down to your skin's needs and your personal preference. Need immediate protection with less concern about white residue? Go physical. Prefer something you can apply and forget? Chemical might be your go-to.

Regardless of your choice, the non-negotiable deal is consistent application. It's not just about avoiding sunburn but preserving your skin's health and youthfulness long-term. So, make it a ritual, and your skin will thank you for keeping those harmful rays at bay!

Examples:

ISDIN Photo Eryfotona Ageless SPF 50 (Tinted. Mineral. Love)

DRMTLGY's Universal Tinted Moisturizer SPF 46 (Chemical. Love.)

DRMTLGY's Physical Tinted Moisturizer SPF 44 (Mineral. Love)

Cōtz Flawless Complexion SPF 50 Richly Tinted (Mineral. New Fav)

Special Mentions:

Let's cover some products you may have yet to hear of and some you can't stop hearing about. Some deserve a place on your skincare shelf while others, well... Spoiler alert: it's not all good news.

Coenzyme Q10 (CoQ10): Imagine this as a protective friend for your skin. CoQ10 acts as an antioxidant, safeguarding the skin from the damaging effects of the sun and environmental pollutants, thus reducing the appearance of wrinkles and fine lines. It's the silent guardian working to keep your skin looking younger. But it has a challenge: CoQ10 is a larger molecule and doesn't mix well with water, so it sits on the skin. If you want to use it, try it in a serum or, better yet, a supplement.

Collagen: It's everywhere, right? Collagen is known as the building block that keeps the skin looking firm, smooth, and youthful. With age, our natural production decreases, and the marketing tells us WE NEED IT to replace what we've lost. Listen up: It shares the same challenge with CoQ10. Because of its molecular size, it cannot penetrate the skin barrier. Moisturize with it all you want, but know it's not getting into the skin to 'build' anything. You're better off with the supplements, but those have to travel through the digestive system, and just eating something doesn't put the active ingredients where we want them. Just be mindful of what you're getting for your money. Remember: Collagen is built and used by the cells. We can do things and use things and take things to help our bodies make it, but slathering it on isn't doing much for us.

Jojoba Oil and Emu Oil: Now, these guys merit your attention! These oils are the hydration heroes, particularly for dry and sensitive skin. Jojoba oil is renowned for being most similar to human skin oil, providing moisturizing benefits and helping control sebum production. Emu oil penetrates deep, offering intense moisture, and has anti-inflammatory properties, making both oils substantial for nourishment and healing.

Copper Peptides: Think of these as the renovation crew for your skin. They help to rejuvenate skin cells by promoting collagen and elastin production, facilitating the removal of damaged collagen and elastin from the skin. They're like the task force that cleans out and strengthens the foundation, vital for skin regeneration and healing.

Green Tea: A soothing soul, green tea comes packed with antioxidants, acting as a potent anti-inflammatory and anti-aging ingredient. It's the calming influence that also protects your skin from environmental stressors. It's generally found in a serum form, and it provides outstanding benefits, but do you know what else does? The Tea Bags! Yup. Just strain them and plop 'em right on your face while you relax. Not kidding.

Methyl Estradiolpropanoate (MEP): This dark horse ingredient is a game-changer for estrogen-deficient skin, particularly during menopause. It's designed to mimic estrogen's beneficial effects, revitalizing the skin by improving hydration, firmness, and elasticity without systemic side effects. Consider it a targeted strategy for managing aging concerns during hormonal changes. I'd recommend talking with an Esthetician or Dermatologist before trying it though. It's shown excellent results in menopausal skin, but be warned, it's expensive. Like, really expensive.

Phew! That's a lot to take in, right? But here's the thing: knowing what works allows you to customize your skincare routine like a pro. It's about creating a symphony that resonates with your unique skin needs and lifestyle. The ingredients that matter are those that align with your skin's needs, are backed by science, and nurture by using them in a routine that you maintain with consistency and awareness. So, let's carry this newfound knowledge into later chapters, where we'll delve into crafting that perfect, personalized routine, shall we?

Chapter 2

I'll Take Mine To-Go

Navigating the world of at-home skincare devices is daunting, with countless products promising remarkable results. And believe me, I've fallen for plenty of hype. Have the overflowing bathroom drawer to prove it. However, the truth is that not all are effective. Shocking, I know. This chapter will cut through the noise, providing clear insights into the devices that genuinely work and are worth your investment.

Red Light/NIR Light Therapy:

In the universe of skincare, Red Light and Near-Infrared (NIR) Light Therapy are the stars that shine bright. And if I had to pick only one device to keep, this would be the hands-down winner. These therapies work beneath the skin's surface, speaking directly to cellular mechanisms that encourage healing and combat aging. But here's where you need to pay attention: not all devices are equal. Your choice lies between panels, hard-shell masks, soft-sided masks, and even single bulbs, each with distinct considerations. If you really want to deep-dive this, I recommend you check out Alex Fergus' website at Light Therapy Insiders: https://www.lighttherapyinsiders.com/. He's the master, but here's the bones of the matter.

Panels: These devices are like broad light canvases, offering extensive coverage. They're ideal for treating larger skin areas, encouraging a more holistic healing process. However, their size might make them less convenient for some users. When choosing panels, it's crucial to select those that emit the correct blend of wavelengths, ideally between 630-680nm for red light and 800-880nm for NIR, ensuring the therapy's effectiveness.

Masks: On the other side, we have the more futuristic-looking masks. These fit directly onto your face, targeting the skin with precision, which is perfect for addressing specific facial concerns like wrinkles, rosacea, or acne. Their direct contact allows for intense treatment, but the limited coverage means they're less versatile than panels. Again, the key is in the wavelengths - ensure your mask operates within the optimal range for the results you seek.

The crux of Red Light/NIR therapy lies in consistency and proper usage. The correct wavelengths are non-negotiable, as they dictate how deeply the light penetrates your skin, influencing everything from collagen production to cellular repair. Regardless of your choice, these therapies require time - think of them as a slow, steady journey rather than a quick sprint to the finish line. By understanding these nuances, you equip yourself with the power to reverse time's touch and bring forth skin that tells a story of health and vitality. Using these devices regularly can lead to visible rejuvenation, making them a worthwhile addition to your skincare routine. I use a desktop panel and a soft-sided mask with an additional neck/chest attachment. Honestly, I prefer the panel. I use the mask when I'm absolutely strapped for time and need to move around a bit, but it is a hassle. Plus, the masks just aren't as powerful as the panels. Those are my two cents...

Radio Frequency:

When it comes to advanced skincare, radio frequency (RF) stands out as a revolutionary force. This sophisticated technology harnesses the power of RF waves to penetrate deep into the skin's layers without any surgical intrusion. The magic lies in the energy these waves deliver, warming the skin's tissues to stimulate collagen and elastin production - the building blocks of supple, youthful skin.

Here are the noteworthy benefits and actions of RF therapy:

Tightening and Smoothing: As RF waves warm the tissues, they encourage the skin's natural regeneration process. The result? A noticeable tightening effect, as if your skin's been lifted and smoothed from within. This is particularly beneficial for reducing the appearance of fine lines and wrinkles.

Contour Refinement: Beyond smoothing, RF uniquely helps redefine your facial contours. Hello, jowls! By promoting collagen realignment, it subtly reshapes the skin's surface, perfect for those areas prone to sagging or loss of definition.

Enhanced Circulation: RF therapy isn't just surface-level. The heat generated within the skin boosts circulation, ensuring an increased supply of nutrients and oxygen to your skin cells. This improvement contributes to a healthy, radiant glow, making your skin not just look better but truly feel better.

Safe for Most Skin Types: A stand-out feature of RF is its safety profile. The treatment is generally gentle, non-invasive, and suitable for a wide range of skin types, including those who may be sensitive to more aggressive procedures.

The genius of radio frequency therapy lies in its ability to achieve profound results with minimal discomfort and no downtime. As a matter of fact, I love the gentle heat on my face and neck! It's a cornerstone technology for those pursuing firmer, rejuvenated skin, reflecting the beauty of youth without the tell-tale signs of an artificial intervention.

Examples:
Newa Wrinkle Reduction Device ($$$)
Tripollar - they have several models ($$$-$$$$)

Microcurrent:

In the realm of non-invasive aesthetic enhancement, microcurrent technology emerges as a subtle yet powerful ally. This treatment involves delivering low-voltage electrical currents (hence 'micro') into the skin, which mirror your body's electrical frequencies. These imperceptible currents work to stimulate the muscles beneath the skin, essentially providing them with a 'workout' that helps to tone and tighten.

Here's how microcurrent therapy benefits your skin and why it's become a go-to strategy for maintaining a youthful visage:

Muscle Toning and Firming: Just as exercise tones the body, microcurrent fortifies the facial muscles. The gentle electricity stimulates the muscle fibers, enhancing elasticity and strength. This leads to an improved, more lifted facial contour and a reduced appearance of sagging skin.

Enhanced Collagen and Elastin Production: The electrical stimulation doesn't just stop at the muscles; it also reaches the skin's layers, prompting fibroblasts to ramp up collagen and elastin production. These proteins are vital for maintaining the skin's bounce and resilience, combating the typical signs of aging.

Increased Cellular Activity: By recharging the cells with energy, microcurrent therapy assists in the optimization of their function. This helps in better nutrient absorption, waste removal, and overall skin cell health, resulting in a brighter, more youthful complexion.

Reduced Appearance of Fine Lines and Wrinkles: Through the cumulative benefits of muscle toning, increased protein production, and enhanced cellular function, microcurrent therapy effectively reduces the visibility of fine lines and wrinkles, giving the skin a smoother aspect.

Microcurrent is probably my favorite handheld device. It can be intense or subtle, depending on the treatment selected. Still, I always genuinely enjoy it and look forward to the experience. There is an immediate improvement in the condition of my skin, and also a cumulative one.

Examples:

NuFace

ZIIP

Microneedling: Nano, Cosmetic, and Medical Depths

First of all, YOU CAN DO THIS! There are hundreds and hundreds of videos on YouTube that will walk you through the process, and during COVID, I watched them all. Microneedling is a process that triggers the skin's natural ability to heal and renew itself. The devices, either a 'pen' or roller, use a series of tiny, sterile needles to create micro-punctures in the skin, prompting a wound reparative response. However, you can't just start sticking needles in your face. (I bet you knew that) It's crucial to distinguish between nano, cosmetic, and medical depths*, as each targets different skin issues with varying intensities. I'm going to break each one down, but if you want the best and most in-depth sources on Needling, your go-to will be "The Concise Guide to Dermal Needling" by Dr. Lance Setterfield. It's a tome!

Nano Microneedling:

Depth: Less than 0.15 mm.

Primary Benefits: Perfect for product penetration, nano microneedling doesn't cause actual wounds in the skin but instead creates micro-channels, allowing serums and skincare actives to absorb more effectively. It's painless and offers immediate enhancements in skin hydration and smoothness.

Use: Enhancing daily skincare efficacy, light hydration boosts, and as a preparatory step for more intensive treatments. And remember the products listed in Chapter 1 whose molecules are too large to penetrate the skin? Here's your ticket!

Cosmetic Microneedling:

Depth: Ranging from 0.1 to 1.5 mm.

Primary Benefits: This depth targets the epidermis, reducing the appearance of fine lines, superficial scarring, and mild texture issues. It encourages collagen production and enhances overall skin radiance with minimal downtime.

Use: Regular skin maintenance, early signs of aging, and superficial pigmentation concerns. It's also suitable for at-home sessions with appropriate devices and precautions.

Medical Microneedling*:

Depth: Between 1.5 to 3* mm, typically performed by healthcare professionals. *I list 3mm because you will see it during your own research. Don't do it at home. Leave this depth to a professional.

Primary Benefits: Reaching the deeper dermal layers, this method treats more severe skin conditions such as deep wrinkles, scars, stretch marks, and significant texture irregularities. It triggers a more robust healing response, resulting in transformative skin rejuvenation.

Targeted treatment plans for complex skin issues, often as part of a broader skin care regimen under professional guidance.

Here's a bit on my own experiences with Microneedling: It works, I love it, and I will continue to use it. It also stings (that means it hurts), but OTC numbing cream does the trick. Now for what I've learned from my own skin: More is not more. You don't 'need to bleed', and deeper isn't better for cosmetic level improvements. Also, I'm cycling six months of microneedling (at cosmetic depths - once per month) with six months of TCA peels (see next section - also monthly) and getting some pretty impressive results.

One more note and we'll move on: Dermarolling. I've tried it, and I continue to use it on my hairline with some results. I do not use them on my face or body anymore because... well, I'm a clumsy idiot and can sometimes slide the dang thing instead of rolling it. That whoopsie leaves a mark!

Chemical Peels: Unveiling Four Front-Runners

Chemical peels are skin problems' worst enemy and your face's best friend. Some work by dissolving the bonds holding dead, dying, and damaged layers so the fresh, healthy layers can make their way to the surface. Others work by penetrating deeply into the pores and are fantastic allies in the fight against acne. Among an array of peels, four stand out: TCA, Glycolic, Mandelic, and Jessner's. Each uniquely alters the skin's biochemistry to reveal the fresh, unblemished layers beneath.

TCA (Trichloroacetic Acid) Peel:

Characteristics: A non-toxic chemical that causes the top layers of cells to dry up and peel off over a period of several days to one week.

Benefits: TCA addresses more serious dermatological issues requiring a deeper peel. It's excellent for treating sun damage, melasma, various types of acne, excessive pigmentation, and surface wrinkles. The process stimulates deeper layers of skin, causing them to tighten and boosting collagen production. Fly away Crows, and take your feet too!

Glycolic Acid Peel:

Characteristics: Derived from sugar cane, this peel penetrates the skin deeply and easily due to its small molecular size.

Benefits: It's versatile, catering to a plethora of skin types and issues. Glycolic acid peels revitalize by exfoliating the top skin layer, diminishing scars, reducing signs of premature aging, and evening out skin tone. It's also a boon for acne-prone skin due to its pore-clearing capabilities.

Mandelic Acid Peel:

Characteristics: Extracted from bitter almonds, this peel has larger molecules, making it less penetrating and irritating than glycolic acid.

Benefits: Mandelic acid peels are gentle and work well for sensitive skin, treating fine lines, acne, and sun damage. It's particularly effective for individuals with darker skin tones, reducing hyperpigmentation risks associated with deeper peels.

Jessner's Peel:

Characteristics: A concoction of lactic acid, salicylic acid, and resorcinol, this solution breaks down the upper layers of the skin to shed away dead cells.

Benefits: Jessner's peel penetrates deeper than AHA-based peels, effectively addressing cystic acne, extensive discoloration, and more pronounced signs of aging. It offers comprehensive resurfacing, leading to smoother, more vibrant skin.

I've mentioned Alex Fergus as my go-to guy on all things Red Light and Dr. Lance Setterfield for Needling. Now, I recommend Jennifer Tilney at Platinum Skin Care for her unparalleled educational videos on Peeling. She has a line of very well-formulated skincare products, too (I mentioned some above). Still, the real stand-out is her entire series, and it's growing every week, of Peel University videos that are just phenomenal - and free.

Wrap it up - I'll take it.

These are the four items that made the cut, and do not collect dust in my linen closet. But let's get real for a minute. They're only going to work if you commit, and I mean really work at using them regularly. And now let's get really real: None of them are going to change your face - for that, (you know this) you're gonna need the doctor. The at-home treatments are a long-term, subtle game. I like them, and I even love some of them, but I've decided to stop with what I have. No more devices. I'll put the money towards a neck lift, and I'll not judge myself for it.

Chapter 3

PUTTING YOUR MOVES TO A GROOVE!

We've talked about the stuff and the tools; now let's talk about...THE PLAN. Nothing will work if we don't first apply the most essential principles: Commitment and Dedication. I know you know this, but let's go over it again: this is the cornerstone of any successful skincare journey. Remember, the skin you're in didn't age overnight. It's been through the high heat of sunny days and the harsh cold of wintery nights. It's seen stressful days and sleepless nights. Unraveling this lifetime of stories etched into our skin layers doesn't come quick—it's a marathon, not a sprint. But with a consistent, dedicated routine, your skin can rebuild and rebound to its (more) youthful days of radiance. In this chapter, we'll work on building your game plans. A simple routine can be as easy as cleansing, moisturizing, SPF, and go. Easy peasy. But since you're here, let's try for at least one more step, okay?

Simple AM:

Cleanse: You did it the night before, so why now again? I get it, I do, and sometimes mine is as simple as a few swipes of micellar water (drugstore stuff, nothing fancy) with some cotton pads. When I have a few extra minutes, I'll use either a mildly exfoliating cleanser or something a little more gentle like CeraVe or Cetaphil.

Toner: This is really up to you. Some experts demand it, others eschew it entirely, and I rarely use it myself. When I do, I use a very mild resurfacing (acids) toner with green tea extracts from Maysama. The two deciding factors for me are: does my skin feel like it needs it, and do I remember I have it.

Antioxidant Serum: This is where your Vitamin C, Astaxanthin, Niacinamide, Green Tea, or other antioxidant serums come in. They really are critical to fighting the free radicals that will be marching their protests across our faces in the hours to come.

Moisturize: My skin tends to feel dehydrated, so I opt for a moisturizer that has a healthy dose of HA - like we talked about earlier. Depending on how dry I'm feeling, I'll follow it up with, or even mix together in my palm, some Jojoba or Emu Oil.

SPF: You KNEW this was coming!!!! If I'm careful around my eyes (I never am and still can't learn), I can use a chemical sunscreen. More often than not (should be always for Dumbo fingers here), I'll grab my mineral sunscreen with tint.

This is my - drinking coffee while putting on mascara and looking for my other shoe while I run out the door routine.

Expanded AM:

When you have extra time or are working on a specific issue needing an additional topical or two.

Cleanse: I don't double cleanse in the morning, so I'll just grab one of the basic cleansers I use regularly - but not an oil base.

Toner: Again, this is optional, but keep it simple.

Vitamin C and Green Tea extracts: Allow to sit for 10 minutes... and the next step is why:

Red Light (panel or mask): Studies are showing that Vitamin C and green tea extracts work in concert to improve the results of red light therapy - but you want them wholly absorbed before going Roxanne and turning on the Red Light.

Niacinamide and any other serum I'm using. This is also where you would use specialized topicals for acne or hyperpigmentation. NOTE: The antioxidants play well together and can be used day or night. However, C doesn't like the exfoliating acids, so I keep my orange juice for breakfast. The only reason I use Niacinamide during the day is because I'm already serum-heavy at night and, you know, one less thing.

Moisturize: Nothing fancy here, but I do take my time and still like to mix in one of my facial oils.

SPF: Yes. Always. Even on days inside.

Evening Routine:

Nighttime is when the magic happens. Our skin, along with our entire body, goes into reparative mode during sleep, and the actives we add to our skincare really get a chance to do their work. A simple PM routine might include a soothing cleanser, replenishing moisturizer, and a dedicated eye cream. However, allowing for an expanded routine unfolds layers of nourishment: double-cleansing, powerful active ingredients, treatments for specific concerns, and luxurious oils that lock in moisture, all working overnight during our beauty sleep.

All I'm really saying is try to make more of an effort in the evening. I get it - sometimes, my extraordinary effort is the makeup-removing wipes and moisturizer sitting next to the bed. But don't be me.

Cleanse: This one really counts. You're taking off the day and everything it heaped upon your mug. If you can, try the double cleansing method. Start with an oil-based cleanser (always use dry hands and apply to a dry face). I use a ton of zinc-based sunscreen and usually a setting spray to keep the tint from transferring EVERYWHERE, and this first step is about the only thing that removes all that heaviness. If I'm doing a second cleanse, I just use the same cleanser that I used in the AM.

Toner: I do use a toner when I'm really taking my time. For this, I'll use a moisture-rich formula and pat it into my skin, really focusing on the lines and dry spots around my mouth and my eyes. Let that absorb for a few minutes.

Treatments: The key to layering your products is to go from thinnest to thickest. Here, you can use your spot treatments for acne or hyperpigmentation. This is also where I add my retinol or Tretinoin products.

Moisturize: I really layer it on here, and I love a good peptide-enriched night cream.

Occlude: Try doing this a few times a week, and I promise you'll thank me for it. The idea is to trap all that goodness into the skin by layering an occlusive as the final step. Try Aquafor, good ol' petroleum jelly, or one of your facial oils.

Note: Almost all of your products will say something like, "Add first after cleansing to dry skin." Well, that would mean everything is first?! Nope, what they really mean is to make sure your skin isn't still wet from the previous serum, lotion, or potion. Wait a few minutes between each step, and you'll be fine.

Bonus: Ever heard of Facial Yoga? Me too, and I really don't know if it does much, but it feels good. I realized after starting a program that it was basically the same thing (same movements) that I'm doing with my Microcurrent, so I don't do 'sessions' of face yoga. My version is smooshing my super moisturized skin around and making outrageous faces. Special, right?

I mentioned using a setting spray earlier and want to explain why. Because my skin is on the dehydrated side, I do love using my facial oils, AND I've never found a foundation that doesn't eventually make my dehydrated skin look even worse as the day progresses. So, for me, it's tinted sunscreen/moisturizer. Also, I use mineral sunscreen, which sits on top of the skin. In other words, my tint transfers. The setting spray saves my shirt, his shirt, your shirt...

Skin Cycling

You've done your research and you've found your Holy Grail items. 'These work! My skin looks great! I love this stuff!' And then a few months later, your skin feels like it's losing its lovin' feeling. Skin Cycling may be your next step.

Think of it like this: you go to the gym, you do the same routine for 6 weeks, and Oh BOY, this is working... but then you stall out. Your skin can go through the same process of adapting to your active ingredients. Next thing you know, the WOW results you loved just aren't there anymore.

Don't get discouraged, and don't throw the baby out. The idea here is REST. Allowing your skin the opportunity to repair itself. Try introducing, slowly introducing, different additives. Switch out one type of HA for the other, or try one of the other Vitamin C formulations. Try Lactic instead of Mandelic.

The Cycling part means having different nights for different actives. Day one could be exfoliation, day two for your retinoids, and the next two days for recovery with peptide and ceramide-rich treatments, and then start your 'cycle' again.

This isn't your everyday routine; it's about tuning in to your skin's needs and adapting as they change. Some days, your skin thirsts for hydration; other times, it might be fighting inflammation or an acne outbreak. Skin cycling involves varying products and ingredients to align with these shifts, encouraging optimal skin health.

At-Home Devices and Modalities

We're talking about when and how to incorporate gadgets and extra treatments into your life - and let's face it, you can spend the cash, but if you're not willing to put in the time, nothing will work while it's sitting on the shelf.

As far as gadgets go, I've tried RF, Microcurrent, Laser, IPL (Intense Pulsed Light Therapy), and LED (Red Light/Near-Infrared Light). The IPL and Laser are gathering dust. Not because they don't work, I'm sure they do (probably) - WITH TIME! And that really was the deciding factor for me. One, I didn't love them the way I do the others, and two, I just wasn't willing or able to devote the time needed to see results from using EVERYTHING! Oh, and let's not forget the cash. There's a "Superior At-Home, Cool Laser" that promises results in as little as only SIX MONTHS! And it only costs $2,000! (You read that right) I promise what it will do, and it won't take six months, is slim your wallet by two grand. I'll talk briefly about each one and let you decide if any or all of them are something you'd like to try.

Radiofrequency and Microcurrent:

I'm lumping these together not because they work the same but because you'll similarly use them. To recap what we learned before, RF stimulates collagen and elastin by delivering heat into the layers of the skin, and Microcurrent activates underlying muscle structure. Each device will come with its own set of instructions and suggestions. My favorite (ZIIP, if you want to know) even has a partner app with timed videos synced to the device that guides you through specific routines. Each recommends three to four days a week for an initial period, then regular upkeep sessions less frequently. But seriously, and again, you have to keep it up!

Note: These devices require a conducting gel, conveniently branded and sold by them. Their own gels are lovely! Also, it is not necessary to purchase their brand. Search for an alternative if cost is an issue, and you'll find options. My RF device has a gel I really like, so I wait for sales and stock up.

Microneedling:

Of the two types we covered, Pen and Dermaroller, I prefer the pen for its precision and ease of use. But don't let my tendency for clumsiness deter you from the roller. It really is simple and effective. Please do some research on your own, looking for the least amount of depth needed to address your specific concerns. A simple Google or YouTube search will provide countless results for easy instruction videos. You will need very clean skin! Use an alcohol prep after you cleanse to disinfect (needles, folks!), and you will need 100% pure Hyaluronic Acid for slip. You never want to drag the needles across your skin, like I have. Ouch.

Once you've finished, gently rinse the slip agent and any dried fluid from your skin and follow up with more HA and a facial oil high in linoleic acids.

Examples:
Grape seed oil
Kiwi oil
Emu oil

Nano - Can be used weekly for product penetration.

Cosmetic - Used monthly for skin issues such as fine lines, wrinkles and skin tightening

Medical - this term gets thrown around and misused. You'll find do-it-yourself guides referring to Medical Needling as anything from 1.5 to 3mm. Listen to me: Thou shalt not use greater than 2mm on thyself. Ever-ith. You 'could' use 2mm needles to address stretch marks or other scars on your belly, your thighs, or hips, but NOT YOUR FACE. Got it? Good.

Red Light/Near Infrared Light (LED):

Panels or masks: the choice is really up to you. This can be used almost daily and is lovely for collagen and elastin stimulation, wound regeneration, sore muscles, you name it. It's terrific and something I try to do nearly every day and definitely when I've just done a microneedling session or a Chemical Peel. You'll want dry skin for this, so if you use one of the green tea serums to enhance efficacy, wait about ten minutes to allow the product to fully absorb. We don't want the light reflecting off of the moisture.

Examples:

Isntree Green Tea Toner

Maysama Green Rooibos Pressed Serum

Staying true to the rhythms of your skincare journey demands dedication. It means not just going through the motions but being present in each step and understanding the "why" behind every product application or treatment. It's about promising consistency to your routine, knowing that each day contributes to visible, lasting changes.

To do this, I want to recommend that you keep a journal. It can be a simple spiral notebook or a dedicated Diary App - that's up to you - but I promise you'll appreciate being able to go back and find what's working. Try to take pictures along the way. The before's and after's will be more than enough motivation to keep up your hard work!

So, here's to putting your moves to a groove, dancing in sync with your skin's rhythm, and savoring the journey towards rejuvenation and radiance.

Chapter 4

Every bite you take is a signal to your body. This directive can lead to glowing, healthy skin or, conversely, to a complexion you'd rather keep hidden. It's a universal truth we often forget: the quality of what we consume is mirrored in our skin's health. This chapter isn't about preaching an unattainable diet but highlighting the usual suspects in our meals that, unbeknownst to us, undermine our skincare efforts. When fat combines with sugar, the end product is called Advanced Glycation End Products (AGEs), which triggers damage to our skin cells. It's time to take a magnifying glass to our plates, identifying what needs to be reduced, or better yet, eliminated, to stop the sabotage from within.

Fried Foods: The consumption of fried foods has long been vilified in the wellness community, and unfortunately, the concerns extend to its impacts on our skin's health and vitality. Delicious but devious, these oily culprits contribute to unwanted breakouts and an oily complexion, not to mention wreaking havoc on your arteries.

When food is fried, especially at high temperatures, a sinister transformation occurs. This process is known as glycation, where the sugar in your bloodstream attaches to proteins to form harmful new molecules called advanced glycation end products or AGEs for short. When AGEs accumulate, they make the collagen and elastin fibers stiff and malformed, a phenomenon directly contributing to the loss of facial firmness and wrinkles typical of aged skin.

Here's where it directly affects your pursuit of youthful skin: these AGEs tend to gravitate towards dermal collagen and elastin, the proteins that keep your skin plump and elastic. Once AGEs latch onto these proteins, they render them stiff and malformed, making the skin look less supple, more wrinkled, and generally aged. Furthermore, the high heat from frying instigates an inflammatory response, making your skin more prone to conditions like acne and psoriasis.

Beyond the surface, the oils often used for frying are loaded with omega-6 fatty acids, which create internal systemic inflammation when unbalanced with omega-3 fatty acids. This situation further exacerbates skin issues, contributing to an aged appearance, and can interfere with the skin's healing process.

So do yourself a favor and be prudent to limit the intake of fried foods and preserve not just your internal health but also the youthfulness and vibrancy of your skin. Consider healthier cooking alternatives like baking, steaming, or sautéing in healthful oils to safeguard your skin's elasticity and overall appearance.

White Bread: High glycemic index? Check. Potential to aggravate your skin and disrupt insulin levels? Also, check. When you consume white bread, you're inviting refined carbohydrates into your system, which have a more profound impact on the aging process than you might realize. These refined carbs are stripped of fiber, vitamins, and minerals, leading to them being digested quickly and causing a rapid surge in blood sugar and insulin levels. This isn't just a concern for overall health; it directly contributes to accelerated aging, particularly visible in our skin.

But the effects don't stop at the skin's surface. Internally, refined carbs stimulate the production of a specific group of pro-inflammatory messengers, which activate the body's immune responses. In the long term, this means an increase in general inflammation within the body, known to affect the aging process by promoting degenerative diseases.

The solution? Cutting down on refined carbs like those in white bread and embracing a diet rich in whole grains can help maintain more stable blood sugar levels and provide vital nutrients, slowing down the aging process and benefiting overall well-being. The switch helps safeguard the skin's structural proteins and combats the inflammatory responses incited by refined carbs.

White Sugar: This sweet fiend can also lead to glycation, and the devil, AGEs! Sugar plays a stealthy but significant role in skin aging, particularly in excess. When you consume more sugar than your cells can efficiently process, the excess sugar molecules combine with proteins in your blood, creating new molecules of AGEs. And again, the trouble with AGEs is that they're detrimental to the collagen and elastin in your skin, the proteins that keep your skin bouncy and smooth.

Cutting back on excessive sugar can help maintain your skin's natural elasticity and robustness. Remember, it's not just about looking good; it's also about keeping your skin healthy and resilient.

Processed Meats: Laden with sulfites and other preservatives, processed meats are a no-go for radiant skin. They can dehydrate the skin and deplete it of its fresh, youthful glow. Processed meats, a convenient but less-than-ideal dietary choice, have a sneaky impact on skin health and aging. These products—like sausages, bacon, and cold cuts—are high in elements that don't favor your skin's natural balance. Firstly, they're loaded with salt, and excessive sodium disrupts your body's water balance, potentially leading to puffiness, bloating, and under-eye bags, contributing to a tired, aged appearance.

But the real culprits here are the sulfites and other preservatives that keep these meats fresh. These substances can trigger inflammation throughout the body, and chronic inflammation is a known enemy of healthy skin. It can accelerate the development of wrinkles and fine lines and degrade the natural collagen and elastin reserves in the skin.

Opting for fresher, less-processed meat options can help maintain your skin's youthfulness and overall health. It's one simple change that could yield results you can see and feel.

Charred Meats: That blackened BBQ might taste heavenly, but it's packed with pro-inflammatory hydrocarbons, which could undo your skin's natural buoyancy and brilliance. Charred meats, while often a staple of barbecues and grills, carry implications for skin aging stemming from the process that gives them their distinctive taste: the charring itself. When meats are cooked at extremely high temperatures or come into direct contact with a flame, the proteins in the meat can undergo changes that lead to the formation of even more, you know what it is, advanced glycation end products (AGEs).

To make it worse, the charring process creates polycyclic aromatic hydrocarbons (PAHs). Those are known carcinogens and can also provoke an inflammatory response in the body. Chronic inflammation is another contributor to accelerated skin aging, as it can promote the breakdown of collagen fibers and impair the skin's ability to repair itself effectively.

In light of this, moderating your intake of charred meats and incorporating alternative cooking methods that don't produce these harmful substances—like baking, steaming, or grilling at lower temperatures—can be beneficial strategies in preserving your skin's youthfulness and vitality.

Alcohol: It's a dehydrator and can cause inflammation. Imbibe with moderation, or better yet, swap out the cocktails for hydrating, skin-loving beverages. Alcohol has several impacts on the skin that can accelerate the aging process. Primarily, alcohol is a diuretic, which means it encourages the body to lose fluids and leads to dehydration. Since the skin requires adequate hydration to maintain its elasticity and plumpness, the dehydration caused by alcohol can result in dry, flaky skin that's more prone to wrinkling and fine lines.

Alcohol can also dilate the blood vessels in the skin, and over time, these blood vessels can become permanently damaged, leading to a flushed appearance and visible spider veins. It has an inflammatory effect on the body, which can lead to puffiness, redness, and breakouts due to the alteration of hormone levels and enlargement of the pores.

Additionally, alcohol can affect sleep quality, and poor sleep is known for its detrimental effects on skin health and appearance, including dark circles under the eyes, uneven skin tone, and reduced skin elasticity. It also depletes the body of vital nutrients and antioxidants, which are crucial for repairing skin damage and protecting against environmental stressors.

To maintain youthful, healthy skin, it's recommended to consume alcohol in moderation and to keep a well-hydrated and nourished body. This involves balancing any alcohol consumption with plenty of water, following a nutrient-rich diet, and getting adequate restorative sleep.

High-fructose corn Syrup & Agave: These sweeteners can mess with your insulin levels more than regular sugar, prompting inflammation and oxidative stress. High-fructose corn syrup (HFCS) and agave nectar, both prevalent in many processed foods and beverages, have pronounced effects on skin aging, primarily through their sugar content. These sweeteners are high in fructose, which triggers glycation. The process that produces AGEs, which, in turn, makes the skin more susceptible to wrinkling and sagging.

Furthermore, a diet high in these types of sugars can exacerbate skin conditions such as acne and rosacea, and the inflammation associated with these conditions can accelerate skin aging. Additionally, excessive sugar intake has been linked to poor overall health and can contribute to imbalances that manifest in your skin's appearance.

For skin health, limiting the consumption of products containing HFCS and agave is advisable, focusing instead on whole foods and natural sugars in moderation to maintain the skin's resilience and youthful appearance.

Excess Sodium: Beware the bloat! Sodium causes water retention, leading to a puffy look and feeling. Cutting back can bring back your skin's natural firmness and glow.

Spicy Foods: For those with sensitive skin, spicy foods can trigger flare-ups and rosacea due to increased blood flow. Moderation is key. Spicy foods, beloved by many for their ability to stir the senses, harbor a less-known impact on skin aging, primarily due to their complex interaction with the body's physiological processes. Capsaicin, the active component in chili peppers that imparts the hot and spicy flavor, can influence the skin's condition in several ways.

First is their role as vasodilators—they expand blood vessels, which can increase blood flow and initially give the skin a more youthful, radiant appearance. However, for individuals with sensitive skin or conditions like rosacea, this increased blood flow can exacerbate redness, irritation, and inflammation, factors known to accelerate skin aging if they are persistent or chronic.

Second, the body's response to hot and spicy foods closely mimics its reaction to physical heat: sweating, slight swelling, and increased activity in the digestive system. Excessive sweating and swelling can lead to enlarged pores, dehydration, and collagen breakdown over time, contributing to skin sagging and wrinkling.

Lastly, for some people, spicy foods can trigger inflammatory reactions or allergic responses, again stimulating an inflammatory process in the skin. As with any source of chronic inflammation, this state can promote collagen breakdown, disrupt the skin's natural repair processes, and speed up the development of signs of aging.

For maintaining youthful skin, moderating spicy food intake and observing your skin's response to such cuisine is advisable. Balancing these foods within a diet rich in anti-inflammatory components can also help mitigate potential adverse effects.

Conscious eating is not about deprivation; it's about making informed choices. Understanding the implications of 'garbage in, garbage out' empowers you to control your skin's health narrative. It's a commitment to favoring foods that fuel your glow rather than stealing it. So, the next time you're faced with a dietary decision, remember: the foundation of beauty is not in your makeup bag; it's in your refrigerator.

The adage "You are what you eat" holds a significant truth, especially concerning your skin's health. In this chapter, we confront the uncomfortable reality that some of our favorite comfort foods are, regretfully, skin's formidable adversaries. Making conscientious dietary choices is not just about maintaining a figure or internal health; it's about holistic well-being, which your skin reflects.

On our mission toward enviable skin, it's not just about the potions and lotions you apply; it's equally about the nutrients you ingest. As we cleanse our skincare routine, so must we purify our diet. Replace these detrimental foods with skin superheroes like berries, fatty fish, leafy greens, and nuts. Remember, radiant skin is nourished from the inside out.

Chapter 5

FINAL TALK

As we reach the final pages of this journey to knowledge, let's reflect on the path we've traveled together. Three years ago, I stood precisely where you may stand now—unhappy with the mirror, bewildered by the mirage of the anti-aging skincare world, a world brimming with promises and potions. This maze seemed to offer a thousand pathways but no clear direction. My goal with this book was never just to point you to the fountain of youth in a bottle or device; it was to help light the path so you could walk it confidently, informed, and empowered.

The ingredients we've talked about—those are your trustworthy guides. They are the compass points leading the way: retinoids, antioxidants, peptides, and the humble yet mighty hydrators. They're not just words on labels; they're your skin's allies, each with a role, a purpose, and a time to shine. I've shared with you the times of day when these ingredients do their best work, how they partner with your skin's natural rhythms, and how to layer them like a symphony where every note has its moment.

And the devices! Oh, the magic wands promising the stars. I've been candid about my experiences, the hits, and the all-too-common misses. I've introduced you to the tools that don't just buzz and light up but actually work, resonating with the deeper layers of your skin to bring out that youthful vibrance.

Remember, though, this book is more than a compilation of advice and recommendations; it's a testament to self-care. We are too often putting ourselves last on the list. Still, I'm here to remind you that caring for your skin is not mere vanity (and what's wrong with a little of that?)—it's a celebration of the person you've grown into, the battles you've weathered and the love you have for the person you see in the mirror.

The skincare journey is deeply personal and can be transformative, not just for your skin but for your soul as well. As you've turned each page and absorbed each chapter, you've been building a routine and a ritual, a moment in your day that's just for you, where you can nurture and affirm yourself. In these moments, we often find the clarity and peace that guide us through life's complexities.

As you apply your serums and creams, remember that each application is a layer of intention, a commitment to the belief that you deserve to feel and look your best. The act itself is as rejuvenating as the products.

It's also crucial to be patient. The most effective regimen is the one you stick with. Results won't always appear overnight, but with consistency and care, changes will manifest. You'll catch glimpses of that radiance, that rejuvenated energy, a little more each day. When you do, remember that it's as much the result of your dedication as it is the efficacy of your chosen products and tools.

I hope the advice in these pages acts as a beacon, guiding you toward informed choices and sparing you the confusion and expense of trial and error. The skincare industry is vast and ever-changing, but the principles of skin health are constant. Anchor yourself to them, and you'll navigate this ocean with grace.

In the end, skincare, like life, is a balance—between science and art, between caring for the self and expressing it. You've armed yourself with knowledge; now it's time to embrace the journey with joy and anticipation.

You are not alone on this path. There's a community, a fellowship of individuals who share your aspirations and concerns. I am a part of that collective spirit, and even as this book closes, our conversation does not. I invite you to continue reaching out, sharing your successes, and discussing your challenges. I want to recommend one such community I found that remains my go-to for all things skincare-related: Penn Smith's Facebook Group. Her website, https://www.pennsmit hskincare.com, has links to her FB group, YouTube Videos (a gabillion Reviews and Tutorials!), Instagram, and more. Hers is a community of like-minded people and is genuinely one of the most caring and supportive groups I've come across. If I have a question, my first stop is the FB group and a quick search. I still can't stump the community!

As you move forward, let this book remind you that your quest for youthfulness is valid and valuable. It's not just about looking a certain way; it's about feeling alive, vibrant, and full of the energy that makes every day a beautiful opportunity to celebrate the wonder of being you.

So, as we part ways in text, I am with you in spirit, cheering you on. I am celebrating every small victory and every moment of joy you find in your reflection. You've started as a reader, but you're finishing as a friend, a confidante on this path to reclaiming your youthful radiance. Carry this knowledge, wield it wisely, and let it illuminate the beauty that comes with each new day and each new layer of skin revealed.

Let's raise our glasses (filled with skin-loving water, of course. Or wine. Wine is fine too.) to the journey ahead, the continued discovery of self, and the radiant days to come. Here's to your health, your radiance, and the vibrant life you're living, inside and out.

And remember, in the grand narrative of your life, this chapter on skincare is just one facet of your incredible story. Make it a chapter of joy, empowerment, and self-love. After all, that is the truest form of beauty.

I thank you deeply for taking this time with me. One of my passions is research and sharing what I've learned, and this book has been a heartfelt outpouring of that love.

Most sincerely,

Shanna Getto

References

Barrie, L. et al. (2022) What is 'skin cycling,' and should you try it?, EverydayHealth.com. Available at: https://www.everydayhealth.com/healthy-skin/what-is-skin-cycling-and-should-you-try-it/

Cohen, J. (2019) Evaluation of efficacy of a skin care regimen containing methyl estradiolpropanoate (MEP) for treating estrogen deficient skin, Journal of drugs in dermatology : JDD. Available at: https://pubmed.ncbi.nlm.nih.gov/31860210/

Fergus, A. (2023) The best budget-friendly red light therapy panel review, Comprehensive Health Articles, Reviews & Red Light Therapy! Available at: https://www.alexfergus.com/blog/best-budget-friendly-red-light-therapy-panel-review

Fergus, A. and Wolbers, B. (no date) Light therapy insiders, Light Therapy Insiders. Available at: https://www.lighttherapyinsiders.com/

Irfan, D. and Muhammad, R.F. (2023) Vitamin C skin benefits - 10 reasons on the list, Marham. Available at: https://www.marham.pk/healthblog/vitamin-c-skin-benefits/

Papakonstantinou, E., Roth, M. and Karakiulakis, G. (2012) Hyaluronic acid: A key molecule in skin aging, Dermato-endocrinology. Available at: https://www.ncbi.nlm.nih.gov/pmc/articles/PMC3583886/

Retinoid or retinol? (2021) American Academy of Dermatology. Available at: https://www.aad.org/public/everyday-care/skin-care-secrets/anti-aging/retinoid-retinol

Setterfield, L. (2017) 'Chapter 5: Treatment Parameters and Protocols for Needling', in The Concise Guide to Dermal Needling. Canada: Acacia Dermacare, pp. 130–133.

Shaw, G. (2014) Anti-aging diet: Foods to avoid and foods to eat, WebMD. Available at: https://www.webmd.com/diet/features/is-your-diet-aging-you

Singh, A. and Yadav, S. (2016) Microneedling: Advances and Widening Horizons, Indian dermatology online journal. Available at: https://www.ncbi.nlm.nih.gov/pmc/articles/PMC4976400/

Smith, P. (no date) A master esthetican's guide to healthy, youthful skin, Penn Smith Skin Care. Available at: https://www.pennsmithskincare.com/

Sherman, P. (2015) Four foods that are making you look older than your age, Anavita Skin Care. Available at: Sherman, P. (2015) Four foods that are making you look older than your age, Anavita Skin Care. Available at: https://www.anavitaskincare.com/blogs/news/16874208-four-foods-that-are-making-you-look-older-than-your-age

www.ingramcontent.com/pod-product-compliance
Lightning Source LLC
Chambersburg PA
CBHW070723260726
48660CB00007B/2695